Table of Contents

Understanding and Managing Food Allergies in Children

7.5. What emergency measures should be in place?

7.6. How can we prevent accidental exposure to allergens?

7.7. What resources are available for support?

7.8. How can we effectively communicate with schools and caregivers?

7.9. What are the long-term implications of food allergies in children?

7.10. How often should we follow up with you regarding our child's food allergies?

7.11. What should we do in case of an allergic reaction?

Understanding and Managing Your Child's Food Allergy: A Comprehensive Guide

1. Introduction to Food Allergies in Children

Food allergy occurs when a person's immune system reacts adversely to something in a food eaten by the person. Symptoms of a food allergy include vomiting, stomach cramps, diarrhea, hives, swelling, eczema, itching or swelling of the lips, eyes, tongue, face, or mouth. Food allergies usually develop when a person has been exposed to a specific food repeatedly. When the body's exposure to that food overwhelms the body's system of defense, food allergy results. In other cases, food allergies develop only if a person has been exposed to a sensitizing agent, such as plant pollen, that the body's mast cells recognize as "similar" to a protein in a food, or while the person is taking certain antacids or antibiotics. A wonderful guide for families dealing with it.

Food allergy is not a minor problem; it is the leading cause of potentially life-threatening anaphylactic reactions in children who may ingest as little as one tiny bite of an allergenic food. Annually, there are 30,000 anaphylactic events, 200 hospitalizations, and 200 deaths due to food-induced anaphylaxis in the United States. This is particularly alarming when one considers that there is currently no cure for children with food allergy. Incredibly, one in 13 of all U.S. children under age 18 now has food allergies, with more than 40% of those children experiencing a severe food-induced reaction. Eight percent of children under the age of three suffer from allergic skin conditions. Clearly, this is not a fringe problem; pediatricians will care for numerous patients with food allergy.

2. Common Food Allergens in Children

A food allergy means a child's immune system overreacts to a specific protein (usually) in a food. There is also another condition (not an allergy) called food intolerance, which can feel like a food allergy but is completely different. With food intolerance, the body has trouble breaking down foods, which can cause vomiting, gas, other belly troubles, and some other symptoms. A food allergy can be mild or very severe. A mild allergic reaction can look like hives (itchy red lumps on the skin), stomach problems, or runny nose. A severe allergic reaction is called anaphylaxis (say: Ann-uh-fih-LACK-siss) and can be deadly if not treated right away. Peanut, tree nut, fish, and shellfish allergies are the ones that most often cause anaphylaxis.

Children allergic to milk often cannot tolerate milk products like cheese or ice cream. Children allergic to eggs often cannot tolerate anything made with eggs. Children allergic to soy often do not like the taste of tofu, which is a meat substitute made from soy.

There are many types of things in the environment that a child can be allergic to, and food is a common thing for allergic reactions. The major types of food allergens in children are milk, egg, peanut, tree nuts, soy, wheat, and shellfish. Most children outgrow milk, egg, soy, and wheat allergies. Peanut and tree nut allergies are less likely to be outgrown and have a higher rate of more severe allergic reactions. Fish and shellfish allergies are usually lifelong.

These allergens are called the most common because they cause 90% of all food allergic reactions. A child can have a food allergy to any food; these ones are just more likely.

2.1. Milk and Dairy Products

Management Tools: It's important to closely monitor all food allergies, with milk allergies requiring particularly close attention. When a child is diagnosed with a dairy or a milk allergy, they may be prescribed an epinephrine auto-injector if their allergy is considered severe. An elimination diet, or a diet that eliminates all dairy and dairy products from the child's diet, may be advised by a pediatrician. You will also be seen by a dietitian or a nutritionist who specializes in food allergies. Monitor food labels for milk in both ingredients and the now required allergen statement. Milk is considered a top 8 food allergen and must be labeled if it is in the ingredients.

Some people with a milk allergy are actually allergic to the proteins in beef and eggs. Symptoms: Many children with milk allergies show signs of an allergic reaction during their first year of life. Children who have a milk allergy may experience these symptoms even when exposed to small amounts of milk or dairy, such as after a mother consumes dairy and breastfeeds. Milk allergy may cause gastrointestinal issues, such as acid reflux, abdominal discomfort, diarrhea, gas, or vomiting. When a reaction occurs within minutes after consuming milk or dairy, young children and some parents will experience symptoms such as hives, nasal congestion, coughing, and tightness in their throat or chest.

Milk and Peanut Allergy are the two most common food allergies worldwide. As peanut is considered the most common food allergen in the United States, many people are unaware that milk and dairy products are equally prevalent allergens in food. As with all food allergies, milk and dairy allergies can be mild or severe based on the individual's immune response. The term "milk" refers to milk produced by cows as well as all other dairy products made from cow's milk. Some people who are allergic to cow's milk are also allergic to milk from sheep, goats, and buffaloes. There are challenges that are only posed to those with a milk allergy, regardless of the severity, that are absent from peanut and other food allergies.

2.2. Eggs

Managing egg allergy: The only way to manage a food allergy is to avoid the foods that cause the allergic reaction. There are many good reasons to avoid eggs if your child is allergic. Children, especially if they are young, could eat eggs or put hands on an egg and have a reaction. Everyone caring for your child should help reduce the chance of accidental exposure. Use the Food Allergy Research and Education (FARE) website for a detailed list of foods and products that may contain these foods. It can be time-consuming and frustrating if you do not take the time to read food labels carefully. Experiment with new simple recipes you can make with your child without using eggs.

Diagnosing egg allergy: After you give a history of your child's symptoms, the healthcare provider will try to determine if the symptoms are associated with something your child has eaten or if they happen only in certain situations (e.g. when you cuddle your pet), and if the symptoms go away after you change something (e.g. remove the pet). Your child's healthcare provider may find out if a food allergy is present in a number of ways. Use this information to help keep eggs out of your child's diet and to help you provide the healthcare provider with useful information.

Symptoms of egg allergy: Most reactions happen soon after an egg is eaten, but a severe reaction can happen a few hours later. Anaphylaxis is the most severe allergic reaction. Symptoms may include any or several of the following: Skin problems - rash, hives, itching, redness of the skin. Respiratory tract problems - sneezing, wheezing, throat congestion, shortness of breath. Gastrointestinal tract problems - nausea, cramps, vomiting.

Egg Allergy:

2.3. Peanuts and Tree Nuts

The oral food challenge (OFC) remains the gold standard for the clarification of peanut and tree nut allergy. As a result, the US National Institute of Allergy and Infectious Diseases (NIAID) published guidelines on when peanut-specific IgE testing should be performed before skin prick test (SPT) or OFC and when SPT should be performed before OFC. SPT is not often performed at the first visit with an allergist. However, evidence does suggest that SPT shows a high positive predictive value (PPV) for both a clinical reaction following OFC and anaphylaxis triggered by trace ingestion of nuts because only mast cell-born tryptase in the skin and the lumen is elevated in someone with a positive SPT. In general, all peanut- or nut-specific IgE test results and blood eosinophil test results should be reported either as traditional units (kU/L or cells/µL) or in the allergy or hospital system normal range for your child's age group, and SPT should also be reported as positive or negative on the day of testing. Sputum eosinophils or exhaled nitric oxide testing can further help to establish that tree nuts and not just pollen have caused the accumulation of allergen-specific Th2 cells in the lungs.

Avoidance is the gold standard for the management of peanut and tree nut allergies. However, tree nuts are versatile ingredients found in many food products, including vegetarian meat substitutes, marzipan, cereals, chocolate, salad dressings, and marinades, so avoidance can be quite challenging for those with nut allergies. Peanuts and tree nuts are also a common cause of severe, life-threatening, and fatal anaphylaxis. Epinephrine autoinjectors and first-aid treatment of anaphylaxis should always be kept with your child if they have these allergies. If your child has one of these allergies, you should also ask your allergist if they need to avoid the other or both. Peanut, alone or with tree nuts, is one of the eight major disclosed allergens required to be plainly labeled on all packaged foods manufactured in the US. A diagnosis of peanut allergy can be associated with lifelong anxiety, depression, and social stigma.

Peanuts are not tree nuts (peanuts are legumes), but people who are allergic to them frequently also have allergies to tree nuts (almonds, Brazil nuts, cashews, hazelnuts, macadamia nuts, pecans, pine nuts, pistachios, and walnuts). Peanuts are the most notorious allergen. One study that focused only on tree nut allergies found that 13% of tree nut-allergic individuals avoided them because of peanut allergy. Symptoms of tree nut allergy tend to be more severe in teenagers and adults compared with children. Most adults who die from food-induced anaphylaxis die from peanut or tree nut reactions.

2.4. Soy

Symptoms of a soy allergy vary from person to person and can include hives, redness of the skin, vomiting and/or diarrhea, stomach cramps, itching of the mouth and throat, chest tightness, wheezing, runny or blocked nose, sneezing, headaches, eczema, lightheadedness, low blood pressure, and loss of consciousness. This variability can make diagnosing a soy allergy difficult. Some children are allergic to soy quite others may tolerate soy oil, lecithin or soybean glycerides which are present in many processed foods. However, you should never give your child anything you suspect contains soy, in any of its many forms. These forms may include ingredients such as edamame, hydrolyzed plant protein or textured and vegetable protein. Because milk protein has a very small molecular weight, the protein from a milk-allergic cow may cross-react with soy. This means that the child with cow's milk allergy may also be soy allergic. For this reason, it is often recommended that children with milk allergies be soy-free at least until their first years.

Allergic reactions to food are common in American children, affecting about 6 to 8% of kids under age five and approximately 4% of older children. Although many foods can provoke an allergic reaction, our new guide focuses on preventing and treating allergies to eight foods that most often cause them: cow's milk, hen's eggs, wheat, peanuts, soy, tree nuts, fish, and shellfish.

2.5. Wheat

Symptoms should all resolve within around 2 hours. Your child will usually be offered the wheat again several times on the same day to ensure the food doesn't cause a delayed reaction. The test may be stopped sooner if your child develops an itchy mouth while eating the food (usually seen when a large challenge portion of protein is eaten) and/or one of the other common food allergy symptoms. Non-IgE wheat allergy can also present with anaphylaxis and seizures, which have included acute encephalopathy. FDEIA is a rare and serious reaction that is triggered from exercise alone or within a few hours of moderate-intensity exercise after ingesting wheat. Emotions, stress, alcohol, non-steroidal anti-inflammatory drugs (NSAIDs), or exposure to extremes of temperature – hot or cold, can act as important cofactors.

Babies may develop eczema after birth, and it is important for these babies, and those with moderate or severe eczema and positive SPT to various foods, to have serum-specific IgE allergy testing. Management strategies for preventing wheat are the same as those recommended for preventing peanut allergy. A wheat challenge should be offered to all children who have never eaten wheat, have carbohydrate-induced reactions and have had recent testing that suggests they may now tolerate wheat, so that the burden of dietary restrictions may be lifted.

The symptoms of IgE wheat allergy may range from mild atopic symptoms to anaphylactic shock, but generally, they are less severe than other food allergies. Your child may outgrow their wheat allergy before they start school (around 5 years of age). If your child is continuing to tolerate wheat-based foods, do not cut wheat or gluten from their diet as this can affect further allergy testing.

2.6. Fish and Shellfish

If a child touches fish or shellfish and then touches their eyes, redness and swelling of the eyes can occur. Children with inner ear allergies can experience inflammation in the ear (otitis) right away or the day after ingesting fish. The primary method to diagnose a fish or shellfish allergy is to talk with a board-certified allergist if possible. If the history and physical examination are typical of an allergy, skin and/or blood tests are performed to determine if allergy-related IgE antibodies are present. Once an allergy is documented, counseling from a registered dietitian with food allergy expertise may help answer specific questions, identify suitable permanent diets, and avoid serious nutritional deficiencies. She can offer menu ideas and suggest lower-risk replacements for the foods that need to be avoided. Cases with severe fish allergies determined by an allergist or allergist lawyer require treatment with a systemic (entire body) epinephrine.

Fish and shellfish allergies are two of the top nine allergens affecting children in the U.S. As adults, fish and shellfish allergies tend to persist in greater numbers than allergies to cow's milk, hen's egg, soy, peanut, wheat, tree nuts, and sesame. The prevalence of fish/shellfish allergies has been reported to be as high as 3% and 4%. Fish allergy is most common in adolescents and adults, while shellfish allergy is most common in children, but not exclusive to this age group. Fish allergies can develop before age 1, but they can also develop in older children. It is theorized that many fish and shellfish allergies may be outgrown.

3. Symptoms and Diagnosis of Food Allergies in Children

The diagnosis of a food allergy based on the reported symptoms must be confirmed by medical tests. Doctors can use an allergen-specific IgE test to detect the presence of specific immunoglobulin E (IgE) antibodies to a suspected food. IgE antibodies are signs of the body's reaction to a substance. A food allergy can also be diagnosed through a series of progressively larger doses of allergens placed under the skin or a blood test to obtain a complete blood count (CBC). For children with certain symptoms, healthcare providers may consider using exclusion and reintroduction of possible allergens to confirm the diagnosis of a food allergy. Getting an accurate diagnosis so your child does not falsely "fail" or "outgrow" the allergy is critical. It is important to get an accurate diagnosis even for a food allergy that seldom causes severe reactions.

Children with food allergies exhibit a wide range of symptoms. Skin reactions are the most common; they include hives, itching, and eczema. A food allergy can also cause bloody diarrhea. Other symptoms include wheezing, coughing, and difficulty breathing. Swelling of the face and extremities is another possible allergic reaction. An allergic child can also be lethargic or fussy. A more serious reaction, anaphylaxis, involves symptoms of dizziness, lightheadedness or loss of consciousness, rapid heartbeat, and a sharp drop in blood pressure. Anaphylaxis causes swelling of the tongue or throat, which can block breathing, and a weak pulse. Most food allergy symptoms occur within 1 to 2 hours of eating. In some cases, symptoms occur in less than an hour. Symptoms may also appear up to 2 hours after your child gets food on his skin or inhales it.

4. Impact of Food Allergies on Children's Health and Well-being

Food allergies may also carry financial burdens. Losing work hours for pediatrician appointments, paying for more expensive foods, and taking time off work to learn how to advocate for children in schools and attend food allergy conferences all have potential dollar impacts. In addition, the lost ability for a child in danger of an anaphylaxis-triggering food to play then live like others carries an immense impact on the family. When a child cannot breathe and break out in hives from a sniff of peanuts or a de-crustified sandwich in a school cafeteria, it is vital to seek out compassion and understanding. An allergy not only affects a child but those around him. Parents and other family members have no doubt experienced abrupt and insecure changes in their lives because of food allergies. What one does about food allergies, however, determines the impact on individuals. While the diagnosis of a food allergy sets limits for all, those who remain in control and face the issues head on might break a cycle of weakened emotional well-being related to it.

The consequences of food allergies. Like many diseases, food allergies have a profound impact on health. What goes unrecognized is their effect on well-being too. Food allergies challenge families both emotionally and socially. Eliminating certain foods from the diet impacts a child's growth and development. Parents must become vigilant food label readers. At social events, parents sometimes refuse a treat or discourage their child from playing at another's house because of the risk of accidental ingestion.

5. Prevention Strategies for Food Allergies in Children

A food allergy prevention study in 2015 showed that babies were 81 percent less likely to develop a peanut allergy when they ate a peanut snack three times a week. This finding is in line with the current advice of the American Academy of Pediatrics, the World Health Organization, and the National Institute of Allergy and Infectious Diseases (NIAID) to introduce common allergenic foods to babies as young as 4 to 6 months of age. The NIAID prepared clear and simple guidelines based on the PBS/Wisconsin Food Allergy Program results called Addendum Guidelines for the Prevention of Peanut Allergy in the United States. These guidelines offer three different workable approaches for families to prevent peanut allergy in their babies. While these recommendations are based on scientific evidence, families should talk to their allergists first to determine what is best for their child. Finally, there is emerging work showing the positive effect of probiotics and prebiotics in peanut-allergic children, which may help heal their immune systems and prevent ongoing or future food allergies. Administering single microbe probiotics to babies in pregnancy and infancy has not been shown to prevent allergic disease.

Prevention starts with understanding of the risks involved. It isn't always known what causes food allergies, but some factors that may increase an individual's chances of developing them include: genetics, food ingredients, food manufacturing methods, poor diet of the mother, and antibiotics. For a family that is considering the best way to prevent food allergy in their child, there are a number of avoidable risk factors to consider. An allergist or pediatrician can better assist with implementing these recommendations. At this time, the most promising advice for managing food allergies in infants relates to early, individualized feeding. Multiple studies have suggested that introducing various "allergenic" (or epi-pen-requiring) foods like peanuts, eggs, wheat, soy, and fish at age-appropriate intervals starting at about 4-6 months of a baby's age and continuing at least weekly through the first year can help to prevent food allergy.

Although every parent wants to protect their child from food allergies, most of the information available on food allergies is in reactive mode—what to do if you accidentally gave your child something that they are allergic to. In other words, the field is focused on treating, rather than preventing, food allergies, which are a response of the immune system to food or food ingredients such as milk, peanuts, or wheat. Below are several ways to prevent the development of food allergies in children, as well as some recent happenings and treatment advice.

6. Treatment Options for Managing Food Allergies in Children

Medical therapy involves four main classes of medication: injectable epinephrine (as an autoinjector), corticosteroids, antihistamines, and omalizumab. Injectable epinephrine is broken down in plasma with a half-life of 3 to 6 minutes; not to be mistaken for inhalational epinephrine, which has a half-life of 10 to 20 minutes. It is important to repeat the dose every 5 to 15 minutes in patients with severe cardiovascular or respiratory symptoms and transport to an emergency medical center. Antihistamines, specifically H-1 antagonists, block the effects of histamine and prevent the receiver cells from realizing the mediator. Histamine is then unable to bind to the histamine receptor on the surface. Immunotherapy for food allergy is an active, draw-out treatment that reduces symptoms and prevents the development of new allergic symptoms for one or more allergens. This involves giving children gradually increased amounts of the allergen so that the body's immune system becomes less reactive to it.

Medical Therapy

The cornerstone of guiding care and treatment in food allergies is avoidance of the trigger. Knowledge and education are crucial for parents and caregivers. Mild reactions may benefit from the use of antihistamines (to quell hives and itching). Severe reactions, especially with respiratory symptoms, should be treated with epinephrine quickly, followed by intravenous administration. All caregivers should have access to injectable epinephrine with a prespecified plan from an experienced physician. Mild reactions may also respond to corticosteroids because they have antihistaminic properties.

6. Treatment options 6.1. General

6.1. Epinephrine Autoinjectors

Epinephrine autoinjectors are life-saving devices, and parents need to know why autoinjectors are used, how to deliver a dose, and why they are such an important part of a food allergy treatment plan. A doctor shows the caregiver or child how to use the autoinjector with a training device. Because children grow, those training devices should be available in all sizes so the doctor can offer a size-adjusted training tool for kids to learn from. The entire explanation and demonstration process usually takes less than five minutes. Children 40 kg (88 lbs.) and heavier can be taught to self-inject with the appropriate training device.

Children suffering from moderate to severe food allergies are advised by their pediatricians to own and carry autoinjectors of epinephrine (granted that there are no preexisting conditions that would contradict such advice). Autoinjectors are slender, pen-like tubes containing one or two doses of epinephrine that are administered quickly into the child's thigh. The medication is absorbed quickly, relieving a wide array of symptoms ranging from swollen lips, vomiting, skin hiving, cough, or rapid breathing in a matter of minutes. Pediatricians and pediatric allergists alike stress the importance for caretakers to carry epinephrine autoinjectors with them at all times, particularly when their children are consuming problem foods and when their children leave home, by which it is meant out of parental supervision.

6.2. Antihistamines

For milder symptoms, such as hives, antihistamines can be given to offer moderate relief from symptoms at the time of exposure to the food allergen. Sometimes antihistamines are given 20-30 minutes before an incidental exposure with a known food allergen, such as for a supervised oral food challenge procedure or during planned skin testing, to slow some allergic symptoms as exposure occurs. Antihistamines may be used for a few minutes to 1-3 (or more) days after a reaction, but longer for reactions that are also being treated with glucocorticoids. Studies find that, on average, by 10 hours after giving a dose of liquid Benadryl through the mouth, it is discontinued in many children due to loss of effectiveness if symptoms persist.

Antihistamines work mainly to antagonize, or block, histamine receptors on cells. When given quickly at the onset of a milder allergic reaction, they can reduce symptoms fairly quickly, sometimes within an hour. Common brand names are Benadryl and Zyrtec. It is important to note that antihistamines are not meant to treat serious allergic reactions and should only be given together with epinephrine as needed. Antihistamines are available as both liquid and pill, dissolve in the mouth or allow swallowing, as well as injection forms for intramuscular use (IM). Like with any medicine given to prevent a reaction, a dose and timing schedule can be individualized by an allergist after a reaction.

6.3. Corticosteroids

Weak evidence shows that a burst dose of corticosteroids administered early in a severe allergic reaction may be beneficial. The few studies that try to tackle this question use different kinds of corticosteroids in different kinds of allergic reactions and in different populations of individuals with differing genetic predispositions, different coexisting diseases and different lengths of pre-treatment with antibiotics and steroid treatments. Results from these studies have not always been in accord. Therefore, the authors of the reviews of these studies recommend that in future studies any response potentially protective in food allergy should be of a kind that will help our understanding and management of the allergy rather than specifically looking at steroids.

Supporting evidence

Corticosteroids dampen down the damaging immune response seen in many allergic reactions. When used for this purpose, they cannot be taken by mouth or by injection. Instead, they must be inhaled as a fine mist that gets into the sensitive lining of the lungs to have an effect. For this reason, inhaled corticosteroids have limited use in managing acute allergic reactions. Fortunately, other treatments are presently available and being developed that are more useful for managing food allergy. However, it is interesting to note that inhaled steroids hold off the development of allergen-induced asthma in very young children who wheeze, and even prolonged twice-daily treatment over periods of up to as many as nine years is very safe. It is an added bonus that such prolonged treatment makes the children who would otherwise have had asthma "grow out of the allergy" more quickly.

The role of corticosteroids in regulating the immune response

6.4.3. Potential benefits Parents of children with food allergies often ask whether their children can ever be cured. Although complete resolution of food allergy is possible for some children, it is very concerning for researchers and allergists, as a small number of children undergoing immunotherapy have died. It is thus paramount that children on immunotherapy undergo treatment in controlled research studies with regular monitoring. Despite these risks, immunotherapy represents the most promising area in allergy treatments, and the most advances are likely to occur in the next few years.

6.4.2. Approach Oral immunotherapy consists of giving tiny, controlled and gradually increasing amounts of the actual allergenic food protein to the allergic child in order to make the person less reactive. It is being studied and used more and more. Oral immunotherapy is currently only performed in research centers because it carries a risk of adverse reactions, including anaphylaxis. Sublingual immunotherapy consists of putting a few drops of liquid containing the allergenic food protein under the tongue. No studies have been performed on sublingual immunotherapy in people with food allergy. The benefits of this treatment are increased amounts of the allergenic food protein can be ingested without as much worry of an allergic reaction, medications such as antihistamines and epinephrine may not be needed to block or stop anaphylaxis, children have been able to eat certain foods that they were previously allergic to, and findings from a few studies have reported sustained unresponsiveness following treatment discontinuation, although not all children sustain the effects of such treatments once the food protein is stopped and more research is needed.

6.4.1. Principle The principle behind immunotherapy is to modify the immune response by desensitizing mast cells or basophils and increasing the Treg:Th2/Treg:Th2 ratio. There are currently two main approaches, oral immunotherapy (OIT) and sublingual immunotherapy (SLIT) that are being explored.

7. Creating a Safe Environment for Children with Food Allergies

Teach your child to refrain from eating foods outside of those provided by you. This is a seemingly straightforward concept, but it can become problematic as your child grows and becomes more autonomous. Minimizing risk by restricting food options to those provided by safe sources is an essential part of the management of children's food allergies. Encourage children to seek the guidance of an appropriate adult if they have questions regarding a meal while in the care of someone else. They should be encouraged to be open about their dietary limitations and questions about the components of prepared meals. Notify the child's teachers and school nurse about the child's allergies, and be prepared to supply safe meals and snacks if necessary. Encourage responsibilities inside the classroom for children who are ready to take them on. Encourage them to ask for verification of any assumed threat food when away from home and to have trusted adults study meal labels. Establishing a safe and nourishing climate for your child is crucial to his or her growth and development. By providing a secure and sound environment for your child, you are teaching your child the values of valid nutrition, positive social contact, and emotional security.

We all experience wide-ranging emotions as a result of a child's food allergy diagnosis, but a strong desire to protect children from adverse reactions typically emerges.

Understanding food allergy risk, empowering them to recognize and avoid allergens, and educating appropriate adults will allow the child to acquire key tools that will enable him or her to make educated decisions concerning supplied food. Parents are then given a triple reward, as they're guaranteed the awareness, information, and training necessary to guarantee the child's safety when they're apart from him or her. Here are some suggestions for building a nurturing food-allergy-aware environment for your child.

Creating a safe and nurturing environment

8. Educating Family Members, Caregivers, and School Staff about Food Allergies

School staff (teachers, principals, school nurses, etc.): School staff should be aware of your child's food allergies. Work with them to keep your child safe. Teach school staff to: Recognize allergic reactions and know what to do in an emergency. Understand the specific food allergies your child has. What reactions can happen? How soon after eating the food do reactions typically occur? How much of the food can cause a reaction? How likely is your child to have a reaction based on past history? Know where medicines are stored and when they expire. Be there when your child needs to take medicine. Encourage your child to participate in activities and include him in the fun by planning alternative activities/foods. Work with school staff to educate your child's classmates about food allergy. Arrange for everyone to participate in educational activities, such as making food allergy posters. This helps the entire school to understand the meaning of the warning label. Teach kids that it's important to help keep their friends with food allergies safe. You and school staff need to work as a team. Open communication is the key to your success.

Family members and caregivers who help to care for the child with food allergies: Everybody who helps to care for your child should know about food allergy. They should know about the treatment plans that you and your healthcare providers have developed. Take the time to teach and reteach them about food allergy. Be sure they understand how serious it can be. Talk about food labels and what to look for on them. Make sure they know how to avoid your child's allergens. Share important phone numbers with them. Show them how and when to use an epinephrine auto-injector. Answer their questions and listen to their concerns. Encourage them to take responsibility and build confidence. Assure them that they are playing an important part in keeping your child safe and healthy.

For a child with food allergies to be safe and secure, many people—both children and adults—need to be educated about food allergy.

9. Nutritional Considerations for Children with Food Allergies

To help your child establish the best possible diet, be honest with sources of confusion, worry, or other concerns you may have during your visit. Have an open and honest dialogue about your child's food and allergy-related concerns during these visits. Those who are willing to understand and work with you and your family are the best choice. Children with food allergies often have a number of food-related challenges. They may require a special diet to treat or prevent symptoms. However, when those essential nutrients are excluded from the diet, children who exclude certain foods are at risk for nutritional deficiency. The goal is to strike a balance between providing an allergen-free diet and ensuring that a diet is well balanced and promotes growth, development, and overall good health for children and adolescents.

With 6 to 8 percent of children being diagnosed with food allergies, there are a number of nutritional considerations that should be taken into account. One of the main goals of managing food allergies is to ensure a balanced diet is maintained while also excluding the allergen. Nutritional adequacy is important during this time of growth and development. It is anticipated that children will develop a normal, balanced, and healthy way of eating when it is necessary to exclude one or more foods from their diet. Children often look towards their family members to serve as role models, in terms of food. Thus, in many cases, the mother is solely responsible for the development of how a child approaches food and developing an idea of what foods are good or bad.

10. Psychological and Social Aspects of Living with a Food Allergy

Children who see their illness as unthreatening are found to adhere to a limited diet less often than their allergic peers. Coping strategies and social support could positively influence the allergic child, making him/her more self-confident or able to accept the limitation. Luckily, most children living with food allergies are appropriately managed by their families and healthcare professionals and can live in their community without prejudice or incidents with their peers. Children and young people grown up with these special alimentary needs are neither more hypochondriac, frightened, sadder, nor more concerned than their healthy peers. Previous psychological research has shown that when allergic children are compared with non-allergic, or the parental reports are regarded, most differences are inconsistent - the only significant finding was that some food-allergic children reported in an interview that they were less socially active than their non-allergic peers. For protective factors, the allergic children's emotional well-being has been found to be mostly associated with the health reports of the mother, and not one's "objective medical health". In other words, such studies have highlighted the importance of the psychological welfare of parents in protecting their allergic child's emotional welfare.

The good news is, having a food allergy is not all about the physical risks. While we must all take care to follow all of the allergen avoidance strategies, we must also think about the cultural, psychological, and social aspects of allergy. Not least of these additions are feelings. Eating and drinking are not just about fulfilling a basic human need; they are very emotional behaviors that affect many of our lives' social aspects. We celebrate with food, offer as a gesture, and often bond with family and strangers alike during a meal. Therefore, dealing with allergens is not just about technical nutritional knowledge but involves larger human aspects. The "stigma of allergy" and some other more general "quality of life" indicators represented a new appreciation of the medical approach to food allergy with relevant interest in the social and psychological social traits. The stigma connected to food allergy is expected, though from that it will restrict the contact with others, or whether it is the fear of potential adverse consequences or even death that lead to disregard towards the allergic person, would be interesting to explore.

11. Research and Innovations in the Field of Pediatric Food Allergies

Donna Giannico and Laurie Lachance were still in college when their personal experiences with life-threatening allergies led them to co-found their startup, Tula PBC. Lachance, 22, is allergic to milk, pork, beef, tree nuts, peanuts, and more, while Giannico, 22, cannot safely consume milk, eggs, tree nuts, chickpeas, sesame, and more. The company earned a place in the University of Connecticut's Werth Institute, which helps promising young entrepreneurs grow their business ideas into actionable plans. Challenging the status quo around food allergies is their main goal. They want to make the allergy world more connected, safer, and better. A changing landscape more entrepreneurs are making waves in the allergy world right now with their trailblazing innovations, holistic platforms, and promising treatments. From drug companies to empathetic startups, for-profit and nonprofit enterprises to global multi-brand corporations, today's leaders are making investments and pledging resources to grow the competitive and evolving landscape of allergy management.

As we journey through the months of 2022, we will be sharing interesting research and innovative treatments for childhood food allergies. This area is continuing to change rapidly, and we wanted to close out last year by providing a good foundation on where the field is at right now. As you scroll through an Allergic Living article from the fall, you'll notice that start-ups and big corporations alike are investing more in allergy management. This article is the first in a series and provides an introduction to tracking the latest research and innovations live. Follow along to learn about future trends, approved treatments, and advances that may not hit the market for years.

12. Resources and Support Services for Families of Children with Food Allergies

Community support is also recommended. Local support groups and educational resources include physical allergist's office news, school information nights, and annual meetings, as well as parental education designed to help the various features of allergic disease management. In addition, food-free play areas or hospital-sponsored events such as "Peanut Tree Carnival" are designed to provide a shelter for their child-free home. Reachable is an aid association for the family of severe allergies, which is not only a good aspect of resources and support but also offers a great variety of resources and resources for families with less time. Readers can join a food-free list for purposeful and tasting snack and lunch ideas. In addition, there are several websites designed to help children and parents manage allergies and food restrictions, including newsletters, religion-specific camps, books, and recipes. Online resources are convenient but should not be used to inform clients, as not all of these resources reflect up-to-date and accurate advice (e.g., outdated websites may argue with the role of the juice in the child's diet).

Selecting resources and support requires advocacy, empathy, and evaluation. Although some organizations are able to provide direct services to the community, many have complex missions that encompass research, education, and policy. In order to secure support for direct services to the patient community, a wide variety of services must be provided. Ideally, the organization will have medical and counseling services that offer annual retreats, conferences, and information riveting seminars.

13. Conclusion and Future Directions in Food Allergy Management

In testing any allergic child, the allergist, the pediatrician, and you will need to work as a team. Treatment recommendations for food allergy vary according to the severity of the patient's symptoms and his or her history with reactions. The goal is to have a child eat as wide a variety of food as possible while limiting possible reactions. Guidelines to help you meet these goals are found in numbers throughout the statement. Research in the effects of allergic diseases on children is ongoing. Changes in health care practice can be expected as new evidence becomes available. Editorial teamwork to present this publication is sincerely appreciated. And we thank you for reading this information written with you and your Mighty team keep food allergy in mind. We ask researchers, parents, and patients to look towards the future when more results are in and we have more answers. For families dealing with the complexities of food allergies, please know that it is the open-mindedness of scientists that one day may prevent us from calling a child one who is affected by a food allergy.

There are many channels through which you can help make a child less allergenic to a food, but this publication is not meant to be inclusive of all of them. It is, however, a guide to what we do know and what we should be thinking about when taking care of a child with a food allergy at the current time. The management of a child with a food allergy is truly a holistic one. It involves both watching for a severe systemic reaction and considering how that child can best grow to be a healthy, well-adjusted adult while living with his proven food allergy. You will need to work out the child's management plan under the guidance of your child's allergist or pediatrician.

Conclusion

Understanding and Managing Food Allergies in Children

1. Introduction to Food Allergies in Children

The increasing prevalence of food allergy in children observed during the past decades is the subject of ongoing medical and scientific research. It is likely due to a variety of factors. Diagnosis of food allergy in research settings often involves the collection of detailed clinical information and physical exam, allergy skin testing, measurement of serum immunoglobulin E (IgE) to suspected allergens, and exposure tests to determine if food brings about a reaction. The general validity and interpretation of the test results in the context of a suspected food allergy should be carried out by a pediatrician or allergy specialist experienced in the assessment of food allergies in children.

A food allergy occurs when the body's immune system identifies certain foods as harmful and reacts against them. Symptoms of an allergic reaction can be mild, such as a rash or hives, and occasionally require medical attention for severe symptoms such as difficulty breathing or repetitive vomiting. As with other allergic diseases, food allergy can have a significant effect on a child's quality of life and that of the family due to dietary accommodations, social isolation, and bullying. Since the symptoms caused by exposure to a food allergen can be serious, food allergies are the focus of considerable public, academic, industry, and regulatory attention.

2. Common Food Allergens in Children

Nut allergies are allergies to tree nuts. Some nut allergies cause cross-reactivity with related allergens, so if a child is allergic to one nut, they are likely to be allergic to other tree nuts. An allergist can help determine a tree nut allergy. However, in some cases, nut allergies may be cross-reactive between different nuts, and the safest course for someone who is allergic to one nut is to avoid all nuts to avoid cross-reactivity, unless advised otherwise by a clinical allergist.

Peanut allergies are more frequently observed in children than adults. Peanut allergies cause severe reactions in sensitive individuals, some reactions requiring the administration of a narrow time window of an EpiPen. Peanut allergies prevent individuals from coming in contact with any food supply chain items that may contain trace amounts of peanuts. The most common way for children to overcome a peanut allergy is to ingest small amounts of peanut protein over a period of time, slowly exposing a sensitive immune system to a certain amount of peanuts.

In children, there are eight food allergens that are responsible for a majority of allergic reactions: peanuts, tree nuts, milk, eggs, fish, shellfish, soy, and wheat. Though there are many food allergens that can provoke an allergic reaction in children, an estimated 90% of all adverse allergic reactions are caused by these common allergens. While any food can instigate an allergy, these allergens are common in that they are likely to provoke an allergic response, which can range in severity from mild to life-threatening.

2.1. Milk

Milk Allergy: 2.3 percent of Canadian children aged 1 to 2 years have a clinically confirmed milk allergy. Prevalence rates vary between 1.3 percent and 7.5 percent in infants and children. Children allergic to milk are less likely to outgrow their allergy, averaging 2.6 years for persistent milk allergy, compared to three years for other food allergies. Allergists report that allergy to milk is the most common food allergy that they see, while pediatricians indicate that milk is the most common food allergen diagnosed with a skin prick test. Milk is used in over 40 percent of allergen tests between ages 0 to 19. Other names for milk on labels: Ghee, a milk derivative, typically found in Indian foods. Artificial butter flavor. Some examples include margarine, butter flavor, and milk product. Which foods are milk most commonly found in? Milk is found in a number of commercial and packaged foods. Always check the ingredient list for milk, milk products, and disguised names. Dairy products: All food and drinks made with cow, goat, or sheep's milk. Note: If a child is allergic to cow's milk, he or she may also react to goat, sheep, and buffalo's milk. Always ask a doctor before offering these milk options.

A food allergen is a protein that triggers an allergic response in the gut and immune system. Eight foods account for about 90 percent of allergic reactions. These foods are known as the "big eight" and include milk, eggs, peanuts, tree nuts, soy, wheat, fish, and shellfish. This document provides information on the top five allergens, responsible for more than 80 percent of all food allergies in children. If one allergen were to be singled out as the number one food allergen in children, it would be milk.

2.2. Eggs

General Information: Egg allergies are common in infants and young children. Unlike some other food allergies, however, egg allergies are often outgrown by a child's fifth birthday. Because allergies can be difficult to manage, managing an egg allergy will be different for each child and their family. A child who is allergic to eggs should avoid all food containing eggs. Be especially cautious of hidden sources of egg in food because many processed foods, baked goods, and breakfast foods contain eggs. Always read food labels very carefully and teach this to your child as they grow. Children who are allergic to egg may also need to avoid eggs used in vaccines, such as those used in a flu vaccination unless managed by a qualified allergist/immunologist.

For those allergic to eggs, the egg white or protein is the component that causes an abnormal response. The immune system can react to an allergen in many different ways, most commonly with hives, swelling, vomiting, headaches, stomach aches, and trouble breathing; in severe cases, anaphylaxis reactions may occur. Children may outgrow an allergy to eggs. Management plans should be personalized and taught by a doctor who specializes in food allergies.

2.3. Peanuts

What makes peanut allergies different? The offending proteins, a bit of a peptide isolated from peanuts, are chemically related to beans and the structurally uninhibited proteins of lentils. That is enough to get the reaction going because they all share a distant common ancestry. Peanuts and nuts belong to separate families, which makes them chemically and structurally unrelated. The stout cell walls of twin peanuts resist quick digestion, permeating the bloodstream with active peanut antigens over a long time period. The difficult proteins governing an allergic reaction are from a novel set of peanuts. Everything allergenic is found in the fleshy part of the peanut. Commercial peanut butter is the whole peanut measured without peels. It contains an undeclared possible trace amount of allergen.

As inappropriate as the term "peanuts" may seem in today's world of food allergies, it must be addressed for its prevalence and spectrum. As you have been informed, a severe reaction is rarely the first allergic response to peanuts. It is generally preceded by moderate ones and then worsens over time. The most frequent reactions are systemic reactions and hives. Anaphylaxis commonly happens during or after having peanuts. Peanuts are unusual for causing such severe reactions. In many cases, 0.5-2% of boys and 0.6% of girls have a peanut allergy. Of these, 20% will outgrow it at 5 years old and 50% at 10 years old.

2.4. Tree Nuts

The final section of the paper will give an in-depth look into different kinds of tree nuts that kids can be allergic to. This may help clinicians and food allergy families to approach allergies in a detailed way. Each nut subsection will include the 10 different kinds of tree nut allergic reactions, though most of the research comes from studies on peanuts. Then, each of the tree nut subsections will give a short background on the prevalence and importance of it, plus the clinical features, and will end with a final paragraph on its flavors, forms, and functions. Research has also been done to see if oral immunotherapy (OIT) can desensitize an allergic individual to a specific kind of tree nut. The new and updated trends and directions that are being researched in oral desensitization will be discussed in that final section.

Tree Nut Allergies: A tree nut is different from a peanut. Tree nuts grow in trees. Examples of tree nuts used often in America include walnut, cashew, almond, Brazil nut, hazelnut, pecan, macadamia, pine nut, and pistachio. The true prevalence of tree nut allergy is still debated, but the widely accepted number is 1.2% of the total US population. Additionally, the tree nut allergen proteins are stable, can remain on surfaces for a substantial time, and can cause life-threatening reactions in some children. There are currently no US Food and Drug Administration (FDA)-approved foods for children with tree nut allergies, and avoidance of tree nuts is currently the best way to prevent a life-threatening reaction for tree nut-allergic individuals.

Around 12% of US children with a tree nut allergy report having more than one tree nut allergy. And while being allergic to peanuts does not increase the rate of being allergic to tree nuts (and vice versa), many people are allergic to both. 37% of Redwood City US children with a tree nut allergy also have a peanut allergy, and 31% of tree nut children who grow out of one of their tree nut allergies grow into a severe peanut allergy.

2.5. Soy

The management framework for managing soy allergy in an individual child includes careful medical history and physical examination to define the extent of allergy, if any; management of allergic children that is based on the allergen(s) to which they are sensitized; the option of at-home or supervised oral challenges when criteria are met as an important diagnostic tool, and the establishment of a food allergy into which medically are enrolled children who do not currently have symptoms on exposure to the allergen, and whose diet is avoiding that allergen. Optimal management includes early and accurate diagnosis of the child's potential for developing soy allergy and regular review of the nutritional factors that can be improved. Expert recommendations should always be sought in relation to nutritional factors of diagnosis and treatment including type, duration, and elimination of any diet, medical criteria for tolerance, the nutritional impact of allergies and the need for any dietary supplementation. At this stage, the use of soy protein as a 'bath' is not recommended in relation to atopic dermatitis, asthma, other atopic conditions, or food allergy.

Most children with a soy allergy outgrow it by 3 years of age. However, recent research using well-characterized soy proteins has highlighted the severity of symptoms with regards to both IgE- and non-IgE-mediated soy allergy and the likelihood of persistence of disease in some populations. It is not clear whether this is due to children not being included in diagnosis of soy allergy when their only symptom is worsening of their atopic dermatitis or because soy allergy is less severe in atopic children. Soy allergy tends to develop in the first year of life; some children who are allergic to cow's milk may also be allergic to soy, although this is less common than in the past. Despite a general acceptance of the potential of severe soy allergy, some professionals working in food allergy have argued that there is hard evidence of inclusion in many published studies of children who did not have severe reactions to soy.

2.6. Wheat

Although IgE, identified using the RAST-CAP FEIA, was present in more than 20% of children in this birth cohort with non-wheat atopic syndrome, the real prevalence of combined clinical and immunological wheat allergy carried through to school age needs to be ascertained through oral food challenge (OFC). 11. Even if the child's OFC was positive for clinical allergy to a limited number of foods, including wheat, in the pediatric age has a severe reaction in some children. Most guilty, egg 5, dairy, and peanut are common food allergens, possibly responsible for severe and recurrent reactions in any individual, especially if the child has other atopic diseases, such as atopic dermatitis and asthma grouped. In this clinical situation, the clinician should not forget to inquire about the possible ingestion or contact with wheat as this has the potential to trigger an IgE-mediated reaction, which also needs a planned clinical allergy evaluation, including OFC, followed when OFC was negative. While the global supply of wheat is increasing, at the same time, the incidence of wheat allergy in some countries of the world may be increasing, although evidence is required to ascertain this.

1. Introduction and definition. The epidemiology and natural history of delayed wheat allergy in children have been well elucidated. Numerous retrospective studies have examined the occurrence of IgE-mediated wheat allergy in children with atopic syndrome, including eczema and gastrointestinal issues, to more than 70%, in some series. Children with atopic dermatitis (AD) and/or a positive

prick skin test (ST) to egg are at greater risk of wheat allergy than children with AD and negative egg ST. 10. Since the Victorian era, the majority of physicians assume that our understanding of gold-standard wheat allergy is the most common food allergy in children from Asia and Europe to Africa and the United States of patients with AD that is more likely to progress in those with gastrointestinal versus exclusively cutaneous disease. Host and environmental factors predisposing to the progression of wheat allergy in children with AD were partially described in our prospective, birth cohort and we now know that delayed wheat allergy is important in children from Ecuador and the metropolitan area of Philadelphia, PA.

- Wheat rapidly emerged as a common food allergen in six-week surveillance as part of the Center for Disease Control and Prevention-supported Food Allergy Research and Epidemiology Network (FARE). Although the epidemiology and natural history of delayed wheat allergy has been well described in children, there are limited large-scale reports of these children. Notable in the results from six weeks of surveillance is the fact that 46% of egg-allergic children have some form of sensitivity to wheat. Moreover, when tolerance to wheat is achieved in egg-allergic children, wheat can be used as a staple in their diets for nutrition and energy.

Ginger Park, T. Quentin Jones, and Jonathan M. Spergel

2.7. Fish

In our allergy clinics, the most common fish allergy was reported with tuna, salmon, trout, and white fish (e.g. shark, snapper). Detailed fish allergen analysis can determine whether two closely related fish species are equally allergenic or not. Contamination is common in retail fish shops from bench surfaces, utensils, fish mixtures, and water used to defrost fish. Fish-allergic patients who are told that a meal is "fish-free" but contains fish oils can produce an allergic reaction. Fish protein is used in the production of some vaccines. This is called an adverse reaction following immunization (ADFI). Research is being carried out in Australia to develop a more rapid blood test for fish allergy. Skin prick tests are important in diagnosing fish allergies.

A fish allergy is not the same as a seafood allergy. Children may be allergic to fish like salmon, herring, and cod but not allergic to shellfish, the group of marine animals which include crab, lobster, prawn, squid, and scallops. In an international study, fish allergy was shown to be typically outgrown in childhood by the age of 7 years. However, the study showed that despite this, many families continued to avoid fish until age 10 because of fear of accidental reaction. Fish allergy appears more likely to be accompanied by severe allergic reactions, and for some children with asthma, fish allergy appears to be a risk factor for life-threatening anaphylactic episodes. In a recent Australian study, 27% of those with immediate fish allergy had experienced a life-threatening anaphylactic episode involving skin, cardiovascular, and respiratory systems. Anyone with a significant fish allergy should avoid consumption of all fish.

2.8. Shellfish

Another substance that could lead to an allergic response is crustaceans such as shrimp, prawns, crayfish, or lobster. White meat fish include haddock, cod, and sea bass, and they are distinct from shellfish, but several react. It is not unusual for a patient to have an allergic effect to both types of fish, despite the fact that these are different. The only treatment for a shellfish allergy is to avoid eating it, so there is presently no cure. Fortunately, if you or your child are allergic to shellfish, you will almost certainly develop a tolerance. It also helps reduce allergy signs and aids the immune system's recovery by consuming a nutritious diet and consulting with a doctor. There are a few ways to prevent an allergic reaction, and a doctor can help you build a plan. When dining out, be very cautious. Many indigenous, Thai, and Northern Vietnamese meals are flavored with fish or shellfish sauce. A person with shellfish allergies in a community of seafood fans may find it impossible to locate a shellfish-free restaurant.

Shellfish are swimming sea animals that have two groups: crustaceans and mollusks. Contact with just a small amount of shellfish can cause an allergic reaction. A shellfish allergy is an immune system response to a certain protein. Shellfish must be easily identified and listed on the ingredient labels of packaged foods. Products processed in a facility that also processes shellfish will often be labeled as such. Anyone with a shellfish allergy should be instructed to avoid eating them, and parents should provide evidence to the person preparing the food that their child has a severe allergic reaction to shellfish. Members of the mollusk family that commonly cause a reaction are snails, clams, and oysters.

3. Symptoms and Diagnosis of Food Allergies in Children

One important part of managing a child with a food allergy is identifying the likelihood of a food allergy. Infants who have chronic upset stomach, vomiting, or loose stools that do not respond to therapies for other common conditions such as gastroesophageal reflux, gastroenteritis, or constipation could have a milk protein-based allergic disorder. Similarly, hypersensitivity reactions to individuals incompletely digesting different types of lactose that are derived from cow's milk may cause similar symptoms. A child with repeated presentations to the emergency department or to a doctor's office showing symptoms such as eczema, with or without wheezing, flushing, hives, or hoarseness and/or throat irritation, especially following the ingestion of cow's milk, eggs, peanuts, tree nuts, fish, or shellfish, should be considered a candidate for evaluation for food allergy. Abnormal lymphocyte proliferation strongly suggests a food allergy diagnosis. Distinguishing between food hypersensitivity and food allergy is based on the patient anamnesis and other in vivo and in vitro tests, which are often used in combination. Testing such as component-resolved diagnosis is now available.

Food allergies occur when the body's immune system identifies a food as a harmful substance and sets off an allergic reaction in response. They are caused by exposure to specific proteins in a variety of foods. It is important to distinguish between food intolerance and food allergy as the two are different and involve their own problems and management. The symptoms of food allergies can differ from child to child, and reactions can occur after eating small amounts of a food to which a child is allergic. Symptoms may not occur the first time a child is exposed to a food. Food allergies can affect the skin, the gastrointestinal tract, and the respiratory or cardiovascular system. Symptoms of food allergy can occur within minutes to hours of a first exposure to a food or up to several days following a food allergen challenge. Food allergies are often described as a "normal response to unusual proteins."

3.1. Common Symptoms

Parents or guardians may notice that certain foods or liquids cause their child to react with one or more of the signs of food allergy, but subsequent exposure may not result in a reaction. In most reactions, symptoms occur quickly, appearing within a few minutes to two hours of consuming the allergenic food. In a few rare cases, however, the symptoms can occur a few days after exposure to the allergen. If you suspect that a food allergy may be developing in your child or have any questions about food allergy and fast facts, seek medical advice.

Babies may also be diagnosed with acid reflux, but if the baby cannot keep anything down, the cause may be an allergic reaction. The mother and other family members should be alert to food allergy symptoms if the baby has canker sores in the mouth, blood present in the diaper, or a red blood ring surrounding the child's anus. If caregivers see other children showing signs of a food allergy, they should begin monitoring their own children for similar symptoms.

Common symptoms of food allergy in a child may include a red rash, hives, swelling of the lips, face, tongue, or eyes, or chest congestion (noisy breathing, sped-up breathing, or wheezing). Parents should also be alert to lactose or milk protein intolerance, which involves symptoms such as diarrhea, small bloody stool, or mucousy stool, as well as vomiting or poor appetite.

Red flags to watch for: knowing the signs and symptoms of an allergic reaction and learning how to manage them can be key in keeping your child safe and healthy. Be aware that others around your child may not notice a reaction. If your child struggles with an ingredient and you are not 100 percent certain that it came into contact with your child, avoid using that product altogether.

3.2. Diagnostic Tests

The third part involves giving the child the greatest chance of receiving only food alleged to cause them an allergy without increasing the risk. Foods that could cause significant life-threatening reactions should not be consumed, and tests aren't always advised at home because of the risk of life-threatening allergic reactions. Similarly, a placebo-controlled oral food challenge is also used to diagnose food allergies. Testing determines a positive result when a critical reaction occurs during an OFC as a scale value. An OFC involves a person ingesting small portions of a food that triggers allergies, with larger portions being fed at set intervals to evaluate the signs and symptoms associated with their own food allergy.

Routine physical examination and investigative testing for food allergies are often not observed in children with food allergies. Rather, food allergies are generally suspected based on a detailed allergy history and clinical examination. In contrast to adults, it is much more difficult to diagnose food allergies in children. The use of investigative tests should, however, further confirm the diagnosis of food allergies, particularly in equivocal situations, and to determine the absence of allergies in the situations. Although there are benefits to blood tests, they necessitate a blood draw and may cause discomfort and anxiety in children. Thus, the second part of the investigative process is skin testing, a simple, widely used, and bloodless method of screening for food allergies. Skin tests likewise serve as the first stage in the assessment process for kids already on the CDL for allergies. Standard skin testing includes testing for the diagnosis of issues such as allergic rhinitis or cat dandruff.

Diagnosing food allergies

4. Impact of Food Allergies on Children's Lives

The other factors are that children with food allergies and/or their families may have to avoid certain foods, and this has implications for health-related quality of life and dietary status. There is, however, not always a direct relationship between whether avoiding a food has direct health consequences or not. However, avoiding foods can also have frequent social and contextual consequences. From an economic perspective, dietary avoidance can be associated with extra health and social care needs, and parents report that the products they might use to help in managing food allergies can be more expensive than standard alternatives. Medical and non-medical direct costs are estimated to be around 1.3% of an annual healthcare budget for countries such as Australia, the UK, and Japan, although this probably does not capture many wider social care and societal costs. Food allergies, therefore, can affect all aspects of a child's life, from the physiological and psychological to the social and financial. Understanding the complexity of food allergies for children requires the development of strategies that can capture their impact at all 'levels' from the individual to the economy, from the health through to the social. In essence, a holistic approach is needed.

Food allergies are complex and can have wide-ranging consequences for children. One effect is physiological – this can range from skin redness and itching to the most severe allergic reaction, anaphylaxis. Emotional or psychological consequences also stem from children's perceptions of how they think others, such as doctors, family members, peers, and teachers, as well as strangers, perceive food allergies. These views inform how they manage their food allergies and might be a barrier to communication. From a parent perspective, pediatric food allergies are associated with mental health-related quality of life.

4.1. Physical Impact

4.1. Physical Impact. The physical impact of suffering from a food allergy is the impact that the diagnosis has on the physical health of a child. It is an area for which there has been the most research carried out. There is no information specific to the physical impact of food allergies in Eagles' syndrome or Barclay's syndrome. The survey of 100 children found that 95% suffered from a variety of physical symptoms as a result of consuming their trigger foods. A quarter of these children were sent to the hospital on a regular basis to be treated for these symptoms. The Anaphylaxis Campaign and Allergy UK surveys were conducted with the parents of older allergic children, and the children answered the survey themselves. All three surveys were carried out with parents for children suffering from eczema and milk allergy as well as allergy only. It is therefore not possible to say that these surveys give a truly accurate reflection of how often physical symptoms occur. Anecdotally, it is not unheard of for a child to die on their first allergic reaction at home. If a first incident is fatal, it is unlikely that any diagnosis would be made. In addition, those surveys were sent to the parents of those who had good access to healthcare since they were more likely to be members of these two organizations or already be receiving treatment at a specialist clinic.

Food allergies can have varied impacts on different individuals. The following sections detail different aspects of food allergies in children. Some of these observations derive from a survey of 100 children with food allergies that made a connection to another survey specifically for children with eczema that was sent to the Anaphylaxis Campaign and Allergy UK, and some are the result of a food allergy survey of 350 individuals carried out by various regional and national newspapers. A small amount is also based on observations of individuals in clinics. It may be assumed that these children are typical of many of the children that are seen in allergy clinics.

4.2. Emotional Impact

Professionals should identify and address the psychological and family implications of childhood food allergies. It is important that children with food allergies are given adequate information and appropriate support to help them deal with the social, psychological, and emotional challenges faced as a result of food allergy. Strategies to help children cope with food allergies include emotional education, bullying prevention programs, individual counseling, and peer support groups. Health care professionals, including dietitians, are in an ideal position to provide information and referral to specialists. Children with food allergies can experience a significant and undesirable impact on their emotional well-being. One such study quantified the scale of this impact in terms of reduced quality of life. It is important that health professionals are aware of these issues in order to effectively support the children in their care.

Unfortunately, food allergies can cause feelings of fear and frustration in children. It is not uncommon for children to feel excluded in social settings where food is present or suffer embarrassment or a loss of self-esteem when taking special food or being labeled 'allergic'. Parents' concerns, embarrassment, isolation, and depression are also common and can be particularly severe in families of children with multiple food allergies or in children who have experienced life-threatening consequences of allergic reactions. It is important for all families to feel confident about the diagnosis, management plan, how to treat any adverse reactions, and to have regular follow-up visits with a health professional who is competent in managing food-allergic children.

5. Management Strategies for Food Allergies in Children

An individual management strategies for a child with a food allergy might include the following: 1) Wealth of correct food and non-food labels and being aware of possible cross-contamination with labelled products: Reduces the likelihood of accidentally ingesting the allergen; 2) Teaching the child what to do if they accidentally eat a food to which they are allergic, including accessing medical care: The need for an emergency action plan and where they will have access to the medication; 3) Learn the signs and symptoms of an allergic reaction: It is super important for educators to be aware of the signs and symptoms and address them immediately. They may need to administer the auto-injector immediately and call 9-1-1.

The first step in managing food allergies is strict avoidance. This requires reading ingredient lists on food and non-food products and being educated on potential sources of the allergen. Most individuals with a food allergy do not need emergency medication to manage reactions, though antihistamine and/or puffer are typically used to manage symptoms of a food allergy once they develop. For more severe symptoms, individuals may need an injection of epinephrine (adrenaline) from an auto-injector device on the thigh, upper arm or buttocks. The auto-injector is used to manage anaphylaxis, which is a life-threatening reaction. If a child has symptoms that are persistent and/or difficult to manage, they should be referred to an allergist for assessment.

5.1. Avoidance of Allergens

Unsafe Foods If you have a food allergy, you should always remember if a food is unsafe for you, you should never eat it. For parents, this can be a stressful task, but through reading labels, preparation, and organization, it gets easier as time goes on and you gain confidence in your ability.

Keep a List At the beginning, you can ask someone to help you list all the foods that could contain your allergen. Watch out for: any word on a label that you don't understand or could mean a food you are allergic to, any food on a menu (at strangers' houses, parties) where you did not watch the foods being made, any meal that has been made with a sauce, gravy, stock, or other flavoring – these can have your allergen in that you may not think of looking for.

Start Common and Stay Common One way of staying clear of a food allergen is by knowing what foods could contain that allergen. Then you can try to always eat the same, 'everyday' food and cut down on how often you are likely to get the food you are allergic to. For example, how many plain toast or bananas do you see walking around? It also can make it easier for family and friends to know that you are safe to eat at certain places.

Read Food Labels This can be a very hard thing to get right. Many foods contain the foods we need to avoid. Read pre-packaged foods. The ingredients list on a packet of food lists what is in it. The label must show if a food has any of the 14 allergens in it. The list might use words like walnuts or tree nuts. Sometimes the label will also have the allergen information in bold, in italics, or underlined on the label of the product. How ingredients will be written will change depending on the brand.

The most important management strategy for food allergies is the avoidance of the allergen. Preventing your child's exposure to the foods that can cause a reaction is the most effective way of avoiding an allergic reaction. In order to be able to do this, it is crucial to understand the nature of the allergen, read food labels, and choose foods very carefully.

In some cases, a trained qualified allergist or healthcare professional who can oversee any rare side effects can perform an oral food challenge. Once a diagnosis is made and a treatment plan has been proposed, information-based therapy involving parent-directed education has been shown to improve coping strategies and reduce anxiety and depression. Therefore, a role for FARE registry is to reach out to people with known food allergies and/or their families. The FARE registry goal is to enroll 5,000 participants in the first year and eventually to 75,000. This approach gives people with food allergies and their families the power to take actions before accidental exposures occur and/or reactions take root. This access will provide the ability to find additional information about one's own allergy via study results in publications after completion and even to be placed within a local in-person or telehealth medical support group associated with their allergy.

Equally important to knowledge of the severity and prevalence of food allergies and symptoms of an anaphylactic reaction is the ability of providers and caregivers to prepare for them. Adults or children who have been prescribed an epinephrine autoinjector must also have an Emergency Action Plan in place, instructing them and their caregivers on when to use an autoinjector and what to do in case it is needed. A plan should be kept with the child, with autoinjectors, and in several other locations such as home, school, the car, and with the responsible adult. Nut and food allergies are considered laboratory confirmed when there is a detection of IgE specificity (either to the whole food or to a component allergen typically found in the allergenic food) or a positive skin prick test to the food or a finding of a food-specific IgE (≥ 0.35 kUa/L).

5.3. Medications

An autoinjector is a medical device that is specially designed for your child to use, and to be used on them in an emergency. Your health professional is likely to train your child to use the autoinjector when they are old enough. It is especially important for older children and teenagers to carry their adrenaline autoinjector with them at all times – it should not be farther than an arm's length away. If you are uncertain which foods are the cause of your child's strong allergic reaction, a health professional will provide full information. Steroids have an anti-inflammatory effect on a child's body and can help to counter the severe and continuing symptoms of some food allergies, especially anaphylaxis. The reaction may be named or called over time. For example, "latex-fruit syndrome" in someone who is allergic to latex and also sensitized to some fruit.

In managing your child's food allergy, the medications often used to maintain or restore their health or reduce symptoms are antihistamines, adrenaline autoinjectors, steroids, and some other newer therapeutic options. Antihistamines can help to relieve mild symptoms of children's food allergies. In cases of severe symptoms like anaphylaxis or a very severe, generalized skin reaction such as widespread hives (urticaria), affecting much of the body, your child should have an adrenaline autoinjector. It can be given in the outer mid-thigh muscle and often brings immediate relief while waiting for the emergency services to arrive. The action of adrenaline can be helped by your child lying down flat with their legs raised, with their back and head also flat.

6. Communicating with Schools and Caregivers

We cannot know and control all the aspects of the environment in which our children will be, so good relationships between schools, childcare and after-school care should be fostered, rather than ordering them what they should do. Other caregivers should be able to give adrenaline for your child if they are looking after them without you. The My Health Learning and Allergy Tools and Action plans is a very useful online free training course staff can do and print these out after successfully completing it. Staff also need to know that eczema sufferers need to be given an antihistamine if they are very itchy, as eczema is a risk factor for allergy. Et al Lancet. In the preschool, try to talk with the children and their parents about allergies and the different food that people enjoy eating. I often tell the story of Anzac biscuits being my favorite as a child and putting them into boxes for the ADF when I was in the Airforce. We must promote understanding. If the child enters school, we recommend a visit from your school nurse and teacher to your preschool to see how your child is there to help them know the best way to care for them.

Communicating with Schools and Childcare

An improvement in our understanding of the mechanisms of food allergy and tolerance may enable us to develop pro-tolerance therapy in the future. For example, there is some evidence that oral immunotherapy can accelerate the development of oral tolerance in certain situations. As our surveillance databases improve, we may be better able to chart the development of food allergy in childhood and use the information to develop more targeted preventative strategies. It will be important for clinician-researchers to keep in mind the significance of accurate diagnosis when documenting the spectrum of food allergy syndromes.

There is a rapidly growing body of evidence that can guide clinicians regarding best practices in managing patients who are concerned that they or their children may have food allergy. We always want the diagnosis confirmed, so see an allergist with demonstrated training and credentials who specializes in allergies. Thinking of diagnosis is essential when considering all the published literature regarding prevention and management of food allergy. If dietary avoidance adds no benefit, we need to diagnose food allergy accurately so we can graduate allergen challenges. There is some literature that shows that a significant number of diagnoses of food allergy, particularly in the community or low-risk populations, are incorrect when looking at oral food challenges, the gold standard.

Future Directions

7. Questions to Ask Your Child's Doctor about Food Allergies

Not sure what food allergy questions to ask your child's doctor? There are plenty of food allergy facts out there, but sometimes the most helpful information comes from the doctor managing your child's care. Next time you take your child to the allergist or pediatrician, simply print these questions and take them with you to the appointment. It's a good idea to jot down any questions that pop up before the appointment, that way you don't forget specifics you want to ask.

1. Will my child ever outgrow their food allergies? 2. What is a food allergy? How is it different from a food sensitivity or food intolerance? 3. My child was diagnosed with food allergies. What can I - and can't I - send to school as a snack or packed lunch? 4. Some family members seem dismissive of my child's food allergies. How can I/we make them understand how dangerous it is for my child to be exposed to the foods that could make them sick? 5. What is the typical course of treatment if my child has a mild allergic reaction to a food? 6. How do I recognize the signs and symptoms of anaphylaxis and when should I use the Epi-Pen with my food allergic child? 7. If my child has a food allergy, is there a chance it will affect their oral allergy syndrome and environmental allergies?

Here are some great questions to get you started when talking to your child's doctor about food allergies:

7.1. What is a food allergy?

The most severe reaction to food allergies is called anaphylaxis, which is a serious, life-threatening allergic reaction that can come on suddenly. It involves many systems in the body, including the skin, respiratory, and gastrointestinal. Signs and symptoms may include itching, hives, swelling, difficulty breathing, collapse, and shock. Symptoms can appear within minutes when the person either ingests, inhales, or comes into contact with the food allergen. Anaphylaxis should be treated quickly with an injection of epinephrine (adrenaline), followed by a visit to the emergency room. A food that can cause this kind of reaction is known as a food allergen. The food that most commonly causes an allergic reaction are cow's milk, nuts, peanuts, eggs, fish, and wheat. Nevertheless, any food can be an allergen.

A food allergy is a medical condition which develops when the body's immune response to certain proteins in food may lead to physical symptoms. When a person who is allergic is exposed to the food, their immune system sees food proteins, which are usually harmless, as bad and overreacts thinking they are harmful. The system creates a group of antibodies called Immunoglobulin E antibodies to combat the food proteins. The next time the person eats or inhales the food proteins, the immune system releases massive amounts of chemicals like histamine to protect the body. These chemicals trigger symptoms that can affect the respiratory system, the gastrointestinal tract, the heart, and blood vessels, or the skin causing itching, hives, or swelling.

7.2. What are the common food allergens in children?

Milk, dairy, and animal products, as well as eggs, are often identified as causing severe allergic reactions in children. Foods such as wheat, soy, dried fruits and seeds, fish, peanuts, and tree nuts are also common triggers. A dietitian or nutritionist can help establish a balanced diet if any of the common allergy-causing foods listed above are to be avoided.

Per the Australasian Society of Clinical Immunology and Allergy (ASCIA), at least one to two in every 100 children in Australia and New Zealand are allergic to peanuts. Similarly, 2 in every 100 children have an egg allergy and 1 in 50 infants have a cow's milk allergy.

Some foods are more commonly found to cause allergies in children than others. By understanding common food allergens, children and their caregivers can assess what is safe for them to eat and what triggers they should be aware of. This will, in turn, help to improve the management and treatment of food allergies at home and outside of the family environment.

7.3. How is a food allergy diagnosed?

The two recent and probably most widely used allergy tests are the experience of the patient and the result of the skin prick test (SPT), and the percentage positive (or specific IgE above a reference standard) to an allergen - 'sp-IgE', which is obtained from a blood sample and assayed using the Pharmacia of ImmunoCAP or Animal Weight. These are specific tests, in that they test the presence of immunoglobulin (E) antibody produced in response to the allergens ingested. The results are usually expressed as positive or negative, and if the result is positive to two or more allergens, it is more likely that the patient has an allergy. However, quite a large proportion of patients are found to be positive in the allergy clinics but are not allergic to those foods, or conversely, have a strongly suspected food allergy but show negative results to the tests. Extensive allergen testing is expensive and is usually reserved for clinical problems or issues that are to some extent specific to the individual, rather than used as a general screening test.

The diagnosis of a food allergy is difficult and sometimes confusing. A correct diagnosis is even more difficult, and this is critical for the management of children with a presumed allergy. The diagnostic process includes the taking of a careful and accurate feeding and allergic history, followed by physical examination and appropriate laboratory tests. The latter are of greater importance, especially in those with chronic illnesses where the history may be negative but the tests positive. Parents concerned about their child's food allergy should discuss their fears with their family doctors. Most patients will be referred to a pediatrician, especially to an allergist, for further investigations because of the complexity and interpretation of the tests. Management and hybrid food allergy are more difficult, and this is when a more detailed and greater exposure history is important. To clarify the diagnosis and 'rule out or 'rule in' an allergy, investigation may include a progressive exposure diet and supervised food challenges, usually in a clinical setting, as well as valid and acceptable tests.

In this section, we discuss the different diagnostic methods and procedures used in children and describe the new technologies for the diagnosis of food allergies. Fall et al. outlined a 5-step diagnostic procedure, which included taking a comprehensive patient history and performing an allergy-focused physical examination, followed by an appropriate dietary exclusion plan and/or food challenge. Since these guidelines were established, new tests and guidelines have been introduced that focus on improving the diagnostic process further.

3. Baked milk or egg into the diet: If a child has an IgE-mediated allergy, it is likely that the child will grow out of the allergy at some point in time. For children with severe eczema and positivity to baked egg or baked milk, baking will also degrade the allergens and allow parents to see if their child can safely consume the food. It is especially useful if they have tested positive on SPT and specific IgE blood tests. Children should reintroduce the food under medical supervision, and if it is safe they should then try to consume it regularly.

2. Epicutaneous Immunotherapy (or EIT) is when increasing microgram amounts of the allergen is applied gradually to the skin via a patch. EIT has been approved to use in the United States Food and Drug Administration, but has yet to be approved in the UK. These treatments have risks and benefits so it is important to seek medical advice in relation to them.

1. Allergen-specific immunotherapy: This consists of administering increasing amounts of the food in question to induce immune tolerance to the allergen. There are two current types of immunotherapy being studied: oral immunotherapy or OIT is when the food is swallowed (usually in a minuscule amount to start off), and sublingual immunotherapy or SLIT, in which the allergy is consumed and held under the tongue prior to digesting the allergen. OIT can currently be performed in private practice, but it is

a non-licensed intervention because the NHS does not yet believe there is enough safety data to be able to perform this treatment. The main disadvantage of this treatment in children is taking it consistently, in the right way, when life might get in the way. OIT should be introduced with a starting dose in an immunotherapy centre.

In order to help with the management of food allergies, some of the treatments being developed and currently undergoing trials are:

7.5. What emergency measures should be in place?

In addition, it is crucial for parents to be told that an individual with a history of anaphylaxis in the past may continue to experience anaphylaxis at various times in the potential, too despite having their autoinjector. A particle dose accidentally ingested set off the reaction. It is still important for parents of anaphylactic children to call 000 immediately in the event of an allergic reaction. Despite the fact that the kid may become ill, the parent will be able to mediate a potentially life-altering circumstance. Whether an aspirator is available, it should be used to assist the child and, if possible, help avoid airway blockage.

Practically everyone who manages, educates, or cares for the children would see a sense in which monitoring for these development approaches is not a proof, but an absolute duty of care. One aspect that is not commonly regarded is the need to be prepared with emergency measures that are needed to assist with allergic reactions to food in children. Anaphylaxis will rapidly evolve, resulting in death if not treated at the first symptoms emerging or soon after. If a parent has an EpiPen, Twinject, or Symjepi administered in the reaction, the first step a physician would take is crucial. This will assist in slowing the progression of the anaphylaxis, thus buying some time for the patient to reach the nearby emergency department and avoiding death.

7.6. How can we prevent accidental exposure to allergens?

Avoid foods that are not clearly labeled unless you are positive about the labeling policy of the country of origin and have not had previous reactions to similar products. As of 2020, China is the only other country with food allergen labeling laws in place, though these laws apply to different food allergens and different labeling formats. In the European Union (EU), legislation states that prepackaged food which contains a substance considered as an allergen has to be labeled according to Annex II of the EU FIC (EU Food Information to Consumers Regulation). For health and safety reasons, parents and children should also adopt the "safe side" method of assuming that food could contain their allergen.

How can we prevent accidental exposure to allergens? Parents and caregivers are the first line of defense against accidental exposure to food allergens for most children. The most effective ways to prevent exposure are through education, label reading, cross-contact prevention, and food preparation activities. The Food Allergen Labeling and Consumer Protection Act (FALCPA) is a U.S. federal law and its implementation regulation, enforced by the U.S. Food and Drug Administration, which applies to packaged foods. Foods packaged after this date must clearly state, in plain language, the name of the food source from which the major food allergen is derived. The law covers all foods whose packaging is regulated by the FDA, which includes all foods except meat, poultry, processed eggs, and alcoholic beverages, and applies to foods manufactured domestically as well as foods imported from foreign sources.

7.7. What resources are available for support?

There are a number of proposed solutions to enhance the care of children with food allergies, including clearer ownership of the guidelines by medical bodies, ongoing education for healthcare providers, enhancing food allergy management by reducing the cost of specialist visits, and increasing the number of allergists or dietitians going through medical training. Growing numbers of parents and caregivers are asking for the option of having an allergy action plan available as a document that can be stored on their phone. Severe food allergies in children and adults critically rely on those individuals around them being well informed about the nature of the child's allergy and how to manage it. It is our stance that this decision ought to be completely removed from the process of living with a potentially dangerous severe food allergy, so that regardless of what flight a person takes and the airline crew they encounter, they know their allergies will be actively managed effectively. As a starting point, it is critical to ensure all individuals involved in an allergic individual's life are confidently prepared to help them manage their allergies.

Even once a child receives a diagnosis, parents and caregivers often do not have access to the level of ongoing support needed to manage food allergies. There are an increasing number of food allergy experts who are pediatricians, allergists, immunologists, and dermatologists who are equipped to provide support to families. Children with severe food allergies are often under the care of a number of different health professionals, and there is increasing recognition that ongoing psychological support is important. Research shows that management of food allergies is likely to be enhanced by the involvement of psychologists, particularly if a child is experiencing anxiety, depression, or distress in response to ongoing food allergy management. Cognitive-behavioral therapy has been shown to reduce symptoms of anxiety and depression in children and adolescents with food allergy. Parents and caregivers are also supported through ongoing healthcare professional contact and support groups, and a support network on Facebook has proven to be an effective source of support.

7.8. How can we effectively communicate with schools and caregivers?

Often, good communication channels with schools and caregivers will extend to other families, even when they are not actively managing another food allergy. To sustain a healthy relationship, use discretion in your inquiries and communications with schools and caregivers to foster goodwill. It is possible that communication patterns will change over time; what works early in the diagnosis may evolve into different behaviors once their children mature. For example, by the time a child experiences puberty, parents may work directly with the school administration and no longer work with classroom teachers. Independent of the child's age, initiating the school support plan with a letter that briefly summarizes major findings and recommended short-term interventions rather than long-term summaries is the most useful.

One equally important point not discussed enough in primary care is how to effectively communicate with schools and/or caregivers about how to prevent and manage food allergies. Is your question or concern urgent or minor in nature? While it is hard to define these terms, it helps the pediatrician to determine your beliefs and feelings about the care of your child. Remember: "I don't know" is a great answer when you are asked a question regarding the upbringing of your child. Independent of the priority, work with your pediatrician to set time frames when you can expect a response in the course of treating food allergies. If you wonder about unclear guidelines, decisions, or test results, this may not demand immediate attention.

7.9. What are the long-term implications of food allergies in children?

Most parenting strategies focus on meeting the child's immediate needs and reducing food exposure. However, children can react negatively to restrictions and constraints. The feeling of not being able to lead a normal life can generate a feeling of injustice in many children. This can often lead to anger and anxiety issues. Family life can also be tense due to this. There may be disputes between parents and children which can spill over into other aspects of life.

After a severe reaction to a food, your child may be more anxious about trying new food or even eating in general. This can be very challenging for them, and they may especially struggle when not in a home setting. It is important to offer as much support and care as possible. Having a food allergy has been found to increase the prevalence of having asthma and other allergic aspects. This is due to the same cells and molecules being involved in all of these conditions.

While it is important to manage the immediate symptoms when dealing with a food allergy in children, it is just as important to consider any long-term implications. It is hard to know the potential long-term implications fully, simply due to the fact that children will react in different ways. However, this information will offer a range of suggestions and advice to help consider the potential effects in the future.

7.10. How often should we follow up with you regarding our child's food allergies?

In addition to office visits, the use of telehealth has been shown to save families time and money while addressing any primary concerns and questions. Regular and open communication between the family and medical professional is crucial to providing the best possible care and support. We can tailor the office visit schedule to meet the individual needs of each patient in a collaborative fashion.

How often should we follow up with you regarding our child's food allergies? We value our office visits with you to have a comprehensive discussion regarding our child's food allergies. The visits are crucial for prescribing treatment, developing an action plan, and addressing the families' needs and concerns. Moreover, by meeting with you, we can help to prevent potential cross-reactive food allergies. However, the need for follow-up office visits will often depend on the individual situation of each child. A child who has been previously treated by a specialist for only a short period of time may need more frequent visits to observe potential outgrowing of food allergies, while children with multiple food allergies and additional allergic diseases usually require more frequent visits. Adversely, children who are very compliant to an allergen-free diet and do not have a history of bad reactions often only require visits every 6-24 months.

7.11. What should we do in case of an allergic reaction?

Parents should demonstrate how to use epinephrine to family members, caretakers, and the child (as developmentally appropriate). Also, parents and the child should wear Medical Alert identification to inform healthcare providers about allergies and to help assure timely, medically appropriate treatment. A pediatric allergist or pediatrician may offer an anaphylaxis or food allergy action plan, on which parents can fill in important information, such as the child's allergens, an emergency contact (besides 911), and the name and number of the child's primary care physician and allergists. Besides helping administer epinephrine in an emergency, all caregivers should also understand how to summon emergency medical help.

If a child has a mild allergic reaction and the symptoms are mild hives, itching at a single area, and/or mild facial swelling, parents may give over-the-counter or prescription antihistamines. If the child develops severe red hives, swelling that extends to other parts of the body, such as the lips or eyelids, or difficulty breathing, this may be anaphylaxis, and parents should give epinephrine and call 911 for ambulance transportation to the hospital. Even if the child has mild or early symptoms, parents can opt to give epinephrine if they are in doubt whether the child is having anaphylaxis. Emergency medical services can assure that a thorough, complete medical assessment occurs at the hospital, rather than in a clinic or doctor's office. Delay in giving epinephrine has been associated with a greater risk of hospitalization or death related to anaphylaxis.